Cortisol Detox Diet Plan

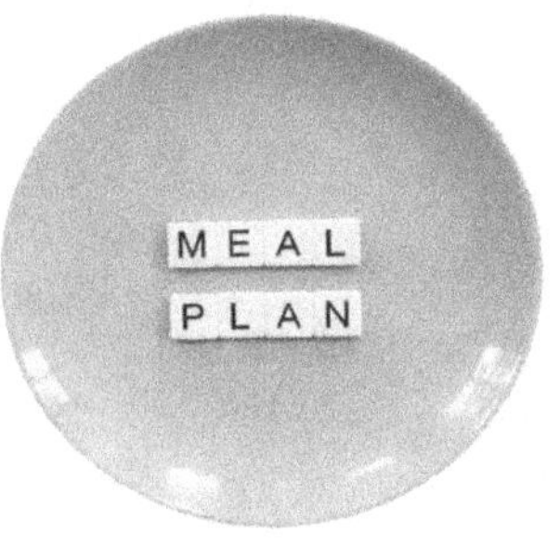

28 Days of Effective Strategies to Manage Cortisol, Reduce Stress, and Achieve Hormonal Balance

~Dr. Sophia M. Wells~

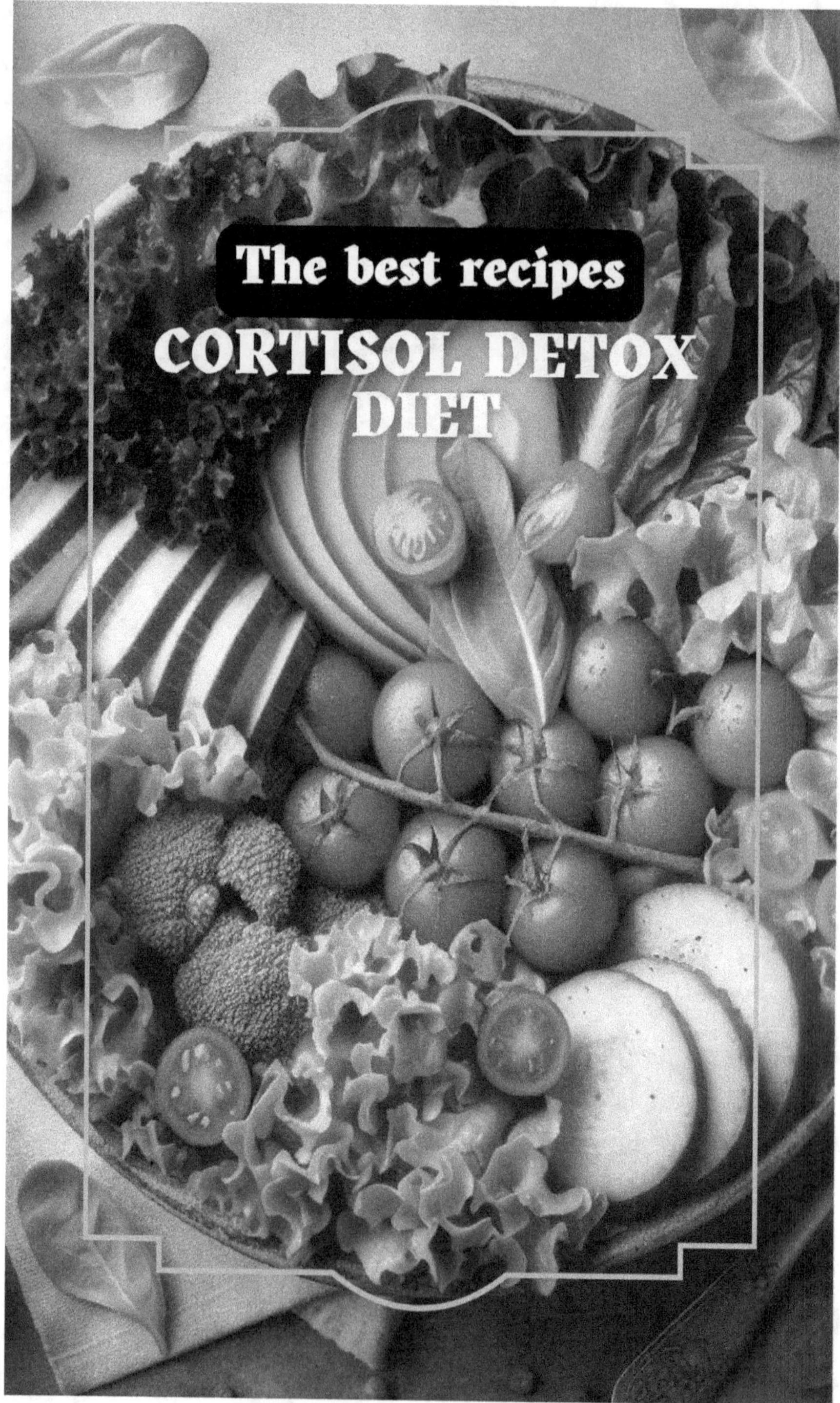
The best recipes
CORTISOL DETOX DIET

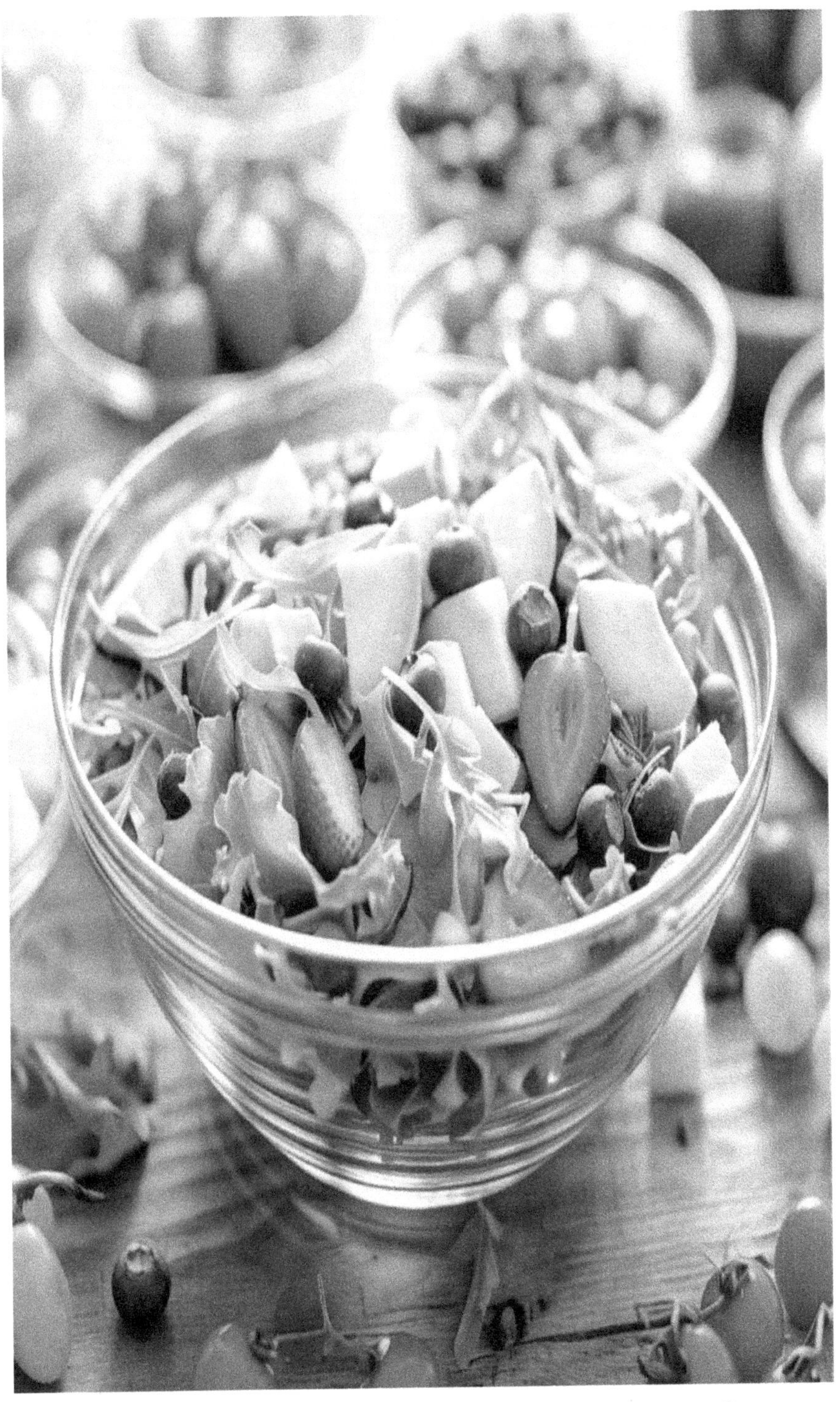

Dedication

To everyone who has ever felt exhausted, overwhelmed, or disconnected from their own peace — **This Book Is For You.**

May these pages remind you that balance is not beyond reach; it's waiting quietly within you.

Acknowledgments

 I want to express my deepest gratitude to every reader who believes that healing begins with awareness and self-care.

To the nutrition experts, wellness practitioners, and scientific researchers whose work helped illuminate the connection between stress and vitality — thank you for paving the way for deeper understanding.

To my loved ones, whose patience and encouragement kept me grounded through every late night of writing — this book carries a piece of your strength.

And finally, to you, the reader — thank you for choosing to begin this journey toward calm, balance, and renewed energy. Your commitment to your well-being inspires everything written here.

TABLE OF CONTENT

Introduction

The Missing Link Between Stress and Your Health

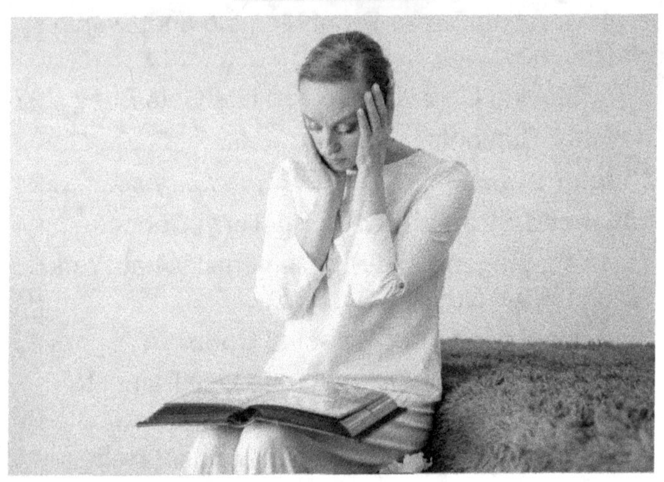

It starts the same way every morning: your alarm buzzes, and before your feet even touch the floor, your mind is already running — thinking of deadlines, chores, or the never-ending to-do list that awaits. You sip your coffee, hoping for energy, but the fatigue never really leaves. Your shoulders tense, your stomach twists, and by evening, even rest feels like another task to accomplish.

If this sounds familiar, you're not alone — not by a long shot. Millions of people wake up each day feeling trapped in this same cycle of exhaustion, tension, and frustration. What most don't realize is that this constant state of overwhelm isn't just "being stressed." It's your body's way of whispering — sometimes shouting — that your cortisol levels are out of balance.

*Cortisol, often called the **"stress hormone,"** is meant to protect you. It's what helps you wake up in the morning, focus during challenges, and stay alert in emergencies. But when life never slows down — when work, family, and worry blend into one long race — your body never gets the signal to rest. Cortisol stays high, silently working against you, draining your energy, fogging your mind, and making it harder to sleep, lose weight, or simply feel like yourself.*

To every reader holding this book right now — the overworked professional running on fumes, the multitasking parent holding everyone together but forgetting themselves, the wellness seeker who's tried every diet and still feels stuck — **this book was written for you.**

I want to start by saying something important: **you are not broken.** You haven't failed your body. You've been surviving in a world that constantly demands more than it gives back. And the fact that you're here, taking this step, means you're already reclaiming your balance — and your power.

This book is your personal guide to healing from the inside out. It's not another diet promising miracles overnight or a list of complicated rules that leave you feeling deprived. Instead, it's a compassionate, science-based roadmap that helps you gently reset your body and calm your nervous system — using the most natural tools we have: **nourishing food, mindful habits, and self-kindness.**

Throughout these pages, you'll learn how cortisol actually works in your body — and how simple shifts in what you eat, how you move, and how you rest can make profound changes. You'll discover flavorful, comforting recipes crafted to lower inflammation, stabilize blood sugar, and support hormonal harmony. Think warm bowls of turmeric-spiced oats on a chilly morning, colorful grain bowls with roasted vegetables and salmon, soothing teas with notes of chamomile and honey, and desserts that taste indulgent yet calm your system instead of spiking it.

Each recipe has been designed with your real life in mind — easy enough for busy days, flexible for all lifestyles, and full of ingredients that taste as good as they make you feel. You'll also find practical cooking tips, ingredient swaps, and serving suggestions that make your kitchen feel less like a chore and more like a sanctuary.

Alongside the recipes, you'll find a **28-day plan** — not a strict diet, but a nurturing structure to help you reset your cortisol rhythm. It guides you step-by-step through balanced meals, self-care rituals, and rest strategies that work in harmony with your body's natural rhythm. By the end, you'll not only understand how cortisol influences everything from your sleep to your cravings, but you'll also have the tools to keep it balanced for life.

And because healing isn't just physical, we'll also explore the emotional side of stress — how to cultivate calm through small, consistent habits. Whether it's setting gentle boundaries, practicing gratitude, or simply learning to slow down and savor each bite, this journey is about more than what's on your plate. It's about rebuilding trust with your body and rediscovering joy in the everyday.

So take a deep breath. You've made it here, and that already matters more than you know. You're stepping into a chapter of renewal — one filled with color, flavor, and vitality. No more chasing impossible perfection or feeling lost in conflicting health advice. You deserve to feel balanced, energetic, and alive — not someday, but starting now.

As you turn the page, remember this: **healing is not about doing everything perfectly. It's about**

listening to your body, one meal, one breath, one moment at a time.

Welcome to the journey. Let's begin your cortisol detox — not with pressure, but with promise. Together, we'll bring your body back into rhythm, your mind back into calm, and your spirit back into joy.

And here's a little tip before we dive in: when you step into the kitchen, do it with curiosity and confidence. Taste as you go. Adjust what feels right. Let cooking become an act of self-care, not another obligation. That's when true healing — and true flavor — begins.

Chapter 1

<u>Understanding Cortisol: The Hidden Hormone Driving Modern Stress</u>

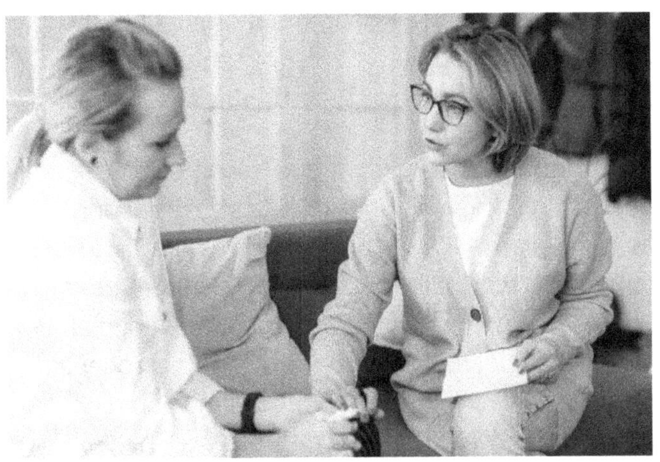

What Cortisol Does in Your Body (and Why It's Not All Bad)

If you've ever felt your heart race before a big presentation, your palms sweat during a stressful meeting, or your mind sharpens in a moment of danger — that's cortisol doing its job. Cortisol is often misunderstood and unfairly labeled as the "bad stress hormone," but the truth is, it's one of the body's most powerful allies when it's balanced. It's produced by your adrenal glands

— small, walnut-sized organs that sit right above your kidneys — and its main job is to keep you alert, energized, and ready to face challenges.

When cortisol functions properly, it regulates blood sugar, reduces inflammation, supports metabolism, and even aids in memory formation. It gives you the spark that helps you rise in the morning and the calm that lets you rest at night. In short, cortisol isn't your enemy; **chronic imbalance** is.

The trouble starts when stress becomes a constant companion. Imagine your body's stress response as a fire alarm. It's meant to go off briefly — to get you to safety. But in modern life, the alarm never seems to stop ringing. Work pressure, financial worries, social media noise, late nights, processed foods, and even constant notifications can all keep cortisol levels elevated. Over time, that "helpful" hormone begins to drain rather than protect you.

How Chronic Stress Keeps Cortisol Stuck "On"

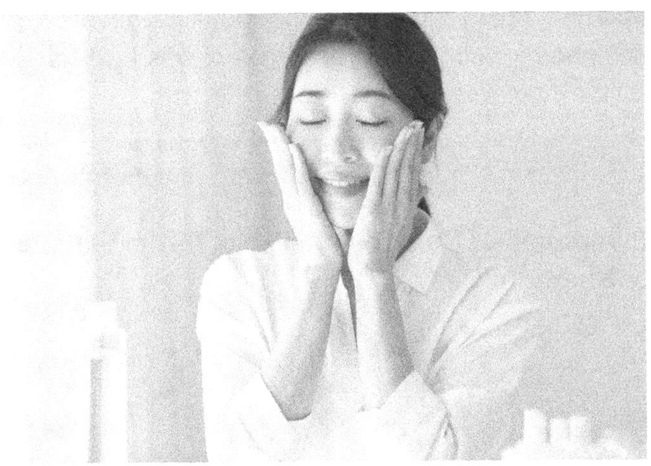

When the body senses danger — whether it's a looming deadline or an actual threat — it signals the adrenal glands to release cortisol. This hormone floods your bloodstream with glucose, giving your muscles quick energy. It slows digestion, suppresses immunity, and sharpens focus — all perfect for short-term survival.

But when that stress never stops, your body doesn't either. The constant surge of cortisol keeps your system in a state of emergency. Instead of restoring balance after the stress passes, your body stays on high alert. This can lead to weight gain, insomnia, irritability, anxiety, and even immune suppression.

The real danger lies in how **subtle** chronic stress can be. Many people don't realize how deeply it affects them until fatigue, bloating, or mood swings become a daily struggle. Your body was never designed for constant pressure — it was built for rhythm, not relentless tension.

Symptoms of Cortisol Imbalance (From Fatigue to Stubborn Belly Fat)

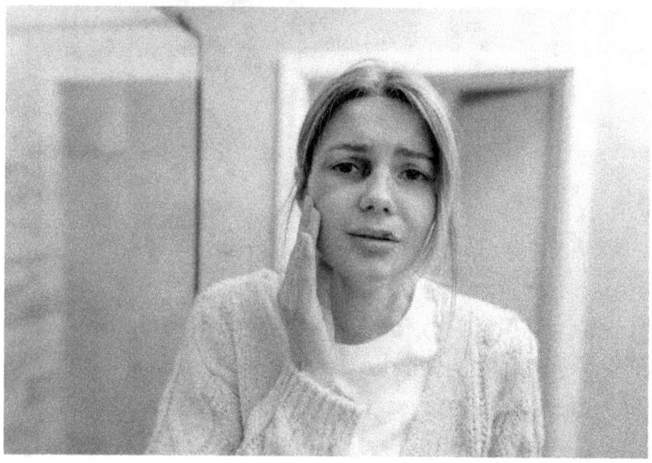

Cortisol imbalance can look different for everyone, but there are telltale signs your body gives when it's overwhelmed.
 You may wake up tired even after sleeping eight hours, crave sugar or caffeine to get through the day, or notice that fat collects around your abdomen no matter how carefully you eat. These are signals that cortisol may be running the show.

Other symptoms may include:

- Trouble falling asleep or staying asleep

- Feeling "wired but tired" — mentally alert but physically exhausted

- Frequent headaches or tension in the shoulders and neck

- Irritability or mood swings

- Poor concentration and memory

- Low libido or irregular menstrual cycles

- Frequent colds or slow healing

These are not random discomforts — they are your body's way of saying, *"I'm overwhelmed."* Recognizing these signs early is crucial to reversing imbalance before it leads to burnout or deeper hormonal issues.

The Science Behind the Cortisol–Insulin–Thyroid Connection

Your hormones are not isolated systems; they work together like instruments in an orchestra. When one is out of tune, the entire symphony suffers. Cortisol,

insulin, and thyroid hormones are three key players
in this delicate balance.

- **Cortisol and Insulin:**
  Cortisol raises blood sugar to give your
  body energy in stressful moments. Insulin,
  on the other hand, helps store that sugar for
  later use. When cortisol remains elevated,
  insulin production also increases to control
  that excess sugar. Over time, this can lead
  to insulin resistance — making it harder for
  your body to burn fat and easier to store it
  around the midsection.

- **Cortisol and the Thyroid:**
  High cortisol suppresses the thyroid gland,
  slowing your metabolism. This is why many
  people under chronic stress gain weight or
  feel cold and sluggish even when eating
  little. A sluggish thyroid means your body's
  natural energy production slows down,
  leaving you tired and foggy.

Understanding these connections is the first step
toward healing. When cortisol finds its natural
rhythm again, insulin sensitivity improves, thyroid
hormones rebalance, and your body begins to feel
lighter, clearer, and more energetic.

How to Recognize Early Warning Signs Before Burnout Hits

Burnout doesn't arrive overnight. It builds slowly —
often disguised as "just being busy" or "a little tired."
But there are red flags your body waves long
before exhaustion takes over.

Pay attention to patterns like:

- Feeling unrested no matter how much you
  sleep

- Mood swings or emotional numbness

- Afternoon crashes or brain fog after meals

- Difficulty losing weight despite effort

- Digestive troubles like bloating or
  constipation

- Losing interest in things that once brought
  you joy

These are early whispers from your body that it's
time to slow down, nourish yourself, and restore
your natural cortisol rhythm.
 When you start addressing these signs through
mindful eating, restorative sleep, and balanced
movement — the same tools you'll find throughout

this book — you can reverse cortisol imbalance naturally and gently.

Lifestyle Foundations for Better Outcomes: Sleep, Movement, and Stress Balance

Food is powerful, but it can't work alone. Your body thrives when your **daily habits** support healing. The foundation of hormonal balance rests on three pillars — sleep, movement, and stress management.

1. Prioritize Restorative Sleep:
 Cortisol naturally rises in the morning and falls at night. When your sleep is disrupted, this rhythm flips, causing fatigue and nighttime alertness. Create an evening ritual: dim the lights, disconnect from screens, sip herbal tea, and let your body unwind. Think of sleep not as a luxury, but as a biological reset button.

2. Move, but Don't Overdo It:
 Exercise helps burn off excess cortisol, but overtraining can push it higher. The key is balance. Combine moderate activities — like brisk walking, yoga, swimming, or cycling — with lighter restorative movement such as stretching or deep breathing. Listen to your body; on tired days, rest is part of the plan.

3. Master Calm in Daily Life:
 Stress isn't going away, but how you respond to it can change everything. Simple habits like mindful breathing, journaling, spending time outdoors, or practicing gratitude can quiet your nervous system. Even five minutes of deep breathing can lower cortisol levels and improve focus.

Final Thoughts

Cortisol isn't your enemy; it's your body's built-in alarm system — designed to protect, not punish. But modern life has pushed that alarm to ring endlessly.
 By understanding how cortisol works, recognizing its warning signs, and building habits that bring your body back into balance, you are taking the first and most important step toward reclaiming calm, energy, and joy.

Every recipe, tip, and daily strategy that follows in this book is designed to help you live in sync with your body again.
 Remember — your body is not broken. It simply needs the right rhythm to thrive.

Chapter 2

<u>The Cortisol Detox Philosophy
Balance, Don't Battle</u>

Why "Detox" Means Nourishment, Not Deprivation

When most people hear the word *detox*, they imagine days of restriction, endless juices, and hunger that borders on punishment. But a true cortisol detox is nothing like that. It's not about removing—it's about replenishing.

Your body doesn't need to be starved or punished to heal; it needs support, rest, and nourishment. Cortisol balance thrives on consistency, kindness, and the steady rhythm of care. Think of this process as a gentle reset—a chance to nourish your cells, calm your mind, and restore natural balance without extremes.

In this philosophy, food becomes medicine—not through limitation, but through abundance. You'll enjoy real meals that taste wonderful, satisfy your hunger, and help your body feel grounded again. The goal isn't perfection; it's progress. Every wholesome bite you take supports your adrenal glands, stabilizes your energy, and teaches your system that it's safe to relax.

Core Principles of Cortisol Balance: Eat, Sleep, Move, Breathe

Cortisol balance rests on four daily practices—simple yet powerful rhythms that teach your body how to find equilibrium again.

Eat:
 Regular, balanced meals signal safety to your body. Skipping meals or eating erratically spikes cortisol levels, leading to energy crashes and cravings. Nourish yourself every few hours with a mix of protein, healthy fats, fiber, and slow carbohydrates. Each meal should leave you feeling calm and satisfied, not wired or weighed down.

Sleep:
 Rest is your body's reset button. While you sleep, cortisol levels naturally drop, allowing healing and hormone regulation to occur. Create a soothing bedtime ritual—dim the lights, avoid screens, and perhaps sip warm chamomile or lavender tea to help your nervous system unwind.

Move:
 Movement is a natural antidote to stress. The key isn't intensity—it's consistency. Gentle exercise such as walking, yoga, or light resistance training keeps cortisol balanced, boosts endorphins, and enhances insulin sensitivity without overstressing your system.

Breathe:
 Never underestimate the power of slow, intentional breathing. Just a few deep breaths can lower cortisol in minutes. When you feel overwhelmed, pause and take five slow breaths—in through your nose, out through

your mouth. It's one of the simplest tools you can use to remind your body that it's safe.

The Four Pillars of Recovery: Nutrition, Mindfulness, Movement, Restoration

The journey toward balance rests on four interconnected pillars that sustain both physical and emotional wellbeing.

Nutrition:
 Food fuels your hormones. The right nutrients regulate cortisol production and help repair the adrenal system. Focus on whole foods—leafy greens, root vegetables, whole grains, clean proteins, and healthy fats. Avoid refined sugars, processed foods, and excess caffeine that overstimulate your adrenals.

Mindfulness:
 A calm mind equals a calm body. Mindfulness doesn't require hours of meditation; even a few minutes of quiet awareness can help. Whether it's gratitude journaling, mindful eating, or spending time outdoors, these moments build emotional resilience and help recalibrate your cortisol rhythm.

Movement:
 Physical activity should energize, not exhaust you. Short, enjoyable routines—like dancing, swimming, or light cycling—improve circulation and mental clarity. Overexercising can actually raise cortisol, so listen to your body's cues.

Restoration:
 Recovery is where transformation happens. Allow yourself to rest deeply—mentally and physically. Take a warm bath, read before bed, or practice yoga nidra. Rest isn't laziness—it's a powerful form of healing that resets cortisol and strengthens your stress response system.

Science-Backed Foods That Reduce Cortisol Naturally

Certain foods have a remarkable ability to soothe your stress response. They stabilize blood sugar, support adrenal health, and replenish key nutrients depleted by chronic tension.

- **Leafy greens** (spinach, kale, Swiss chard) provide magnesium, which calms the nervous system.

- **Fatty fish** (salmon, mackerel, sardines) deliver omega-3s that lower inflammation and regulate cortisol.

- **Nuts and seeds** (almonds, pumpkin seeds, chia) are rich in B-vitamins and healthy fats to steady energy.

- **Fermented foods** (yogurt, kefir, sauerkraut) nurture gut health, which in turn influences cortisol regulation.

- **Whole grains** (quinoa, oats, brown rice) maintain steady blood sugar, preventing cortisol spikes.

- **Dark chocolate**—in moderation—can actually reduce stress hormones and boost mood.

Cooking tip: Try pairing protein with fiber and fat at every meal. For example, scrambled eggs with spinach and avocado toast make a balanced breakfast that supports steady energy all morning.

Key Nutrients for Adrenal Repair: Magnesium, Omega-3s, B-Vitamins, and Adaptogens

Your adrenal glands work tirelessly when you're under stress. To restore their strength, your body needs targeted nutrients that rebuild and protect these essential glands.

Magnesium acts like nature's tranquilizer. It relaxes muscles, improves sleep, and supports over 300 enzymatic processes that regulate hormones. Found in leafy greens, nuts, and legumes, it's a cornerstone of stress resilience.

Omega-3 fatty acids reduce inflammation caused by chronic cortisol elevation. They enhance brain function, support mood balance, and strengthen the body's ability to adapt to stress.

B-Vitamins—particularly B5, B6, and B12—are critical for adrenal hormone production and energy metabolism.

They transform food into fuel and stabilize mood and cognition.

Adaptogens are nature's balancing herbs—plant compounds that help your body adapt to stress. Ashwagandha, rhodiola, and holy basil are among the best-known. They don't block cortisol; they regulate it, helping you find harmony instead of extremes.

Final Thoughts

A cortisol detox isn't a diet—it's a lifestyle. It's about creating a rhythm of nourishment that aligns with how your body naturally wants to function. When you eat with intention, rest with purpose, and move with joy, you begin to build a foundation of calm energy that lasts.

Remember, balance isn't found in quick fixes but in daily choices. With every balanced meal, restful night, and deep breath, you're signaling to your body that it's safe to thrive again.

Chapter 3

<u>Your 28-Day Cortisol Reset Blueprint</u>

Weekly Structure: Reset → Rebalance → Rebuild → Thrive

Transforming your cortisol balance doesn't happen overnight. It's a step-by-step journey, built on sustainable habits that guide your body back to equilibrium. This 28-day blueprint is divided into **four distinct weeks**, each with a clear focus, so you know exactly what to do and why.

- **Week 1 – Reset:**
  The goal is to calm inflammation, stabilize blood sugar, and establish consistent daily rhythms. You'll begin gently detoxing stress-inducing habits like late-night screen time, processed foods, and skipped meals, while introducing nourishing staples to support adrenal recovery.

- **Week 2 – Rebalance:**
  With your system more settled, we focus on fine-tuning hormones and energy levels. This week is about balancing meals, integrating stress-reducing routines, and prioritizing sleep and mindfulness. You'll notice your cravings and

mood swings start to normalize.

- **Week 3 – Rebuild:**
  Now that your foundation is stable, it's time to strengthen your resilience. Focus on nutrient-dense meals, light but purposeful movement, and gentle challenges that push your body to adapt without triggering cortisol spikes. Energy levels begin to rise, and clarity becomes noticeable.

- **Week 4 – Thrive:**
  By now, your system is recalibrated. Week four is about establishing long-term routines, celebrating your wins, and solidifying habits that will keep cortisol in check. You'll notice a stronger immune system, balanced appetite, and a calmer mind.

Detailed Weekly Goals, Emotional Focus, and Food Targets

Each week is guided by **specific goals** — practical, measurable, and achievable — while also addressing your **emotional wellbeing**, because hormone balance is as much about mindset as it is about nutrition.

Week 1 – Reset:

- **Goal:** Reduce overstimulation and sugar spikes.

- **Emotional Focus:** Awareness of current stress triggers.

- **Food Targets:** Leafy greens, whole proteins, complex carbohydrates, hydrating fruits. Avoid processed snacks, refined sugar, and caffeine overuse.

Week 2 – Rebalance:

- **Goal:** Stabilize energy and improve sleep quality.

- **Emotional Focus:** Mindful presence; noticing patterns without judgment.

- **Food Targets:** Include healthy fats (avocado, olive oil, nuts), omega-3 rich fish, magnesium-rich vegetables. Introduce herbal teas and fermented foods.

Week 3 – Rebuild:

- **Goal:** Strengthen adrenal support and resilience.

- **Emotional Focus:** Self-compassion and patience — building trust in your body.

- **Food Targets:** High-quality proteins, complex carbs for steady energy, adaptogens like ashwagandha or holy basil, B-vitamin rich foods.

Week 4 – Thrive:

- **Goal:** Solidify long-term habits for cortisol balance.

- **Emotional Focus:** Celebration and reinforcement of progress.

- **Food Targets:** Maintain a nutrient-dense, balanced diet while experimenting with flavor, creativity, and mindful indulgence.

Step-by-Step Instructions for Transitioning Into the Program

Starting a new health plan can feel overwhelming, but this blueprint is designed to **ease you in gradually**. Here's how to transition:

1. **Prepare Your Pantry:** Remove processed snacks and sugary drinks. Stock up on vegetables, fruits, lean proteins, nuts, seeds, and healthy oils.

2. **Plan Your Meals:** Use the recipes in later chapters as a guide. Choose dishes that excite you, so nourishing your body feels enjoyable.

3. **Set a Daily Rhythm:** Decide on consistent times for meals, movement, and sleep. Consistency signals safety to your nervous system.

4. **Begin Small:** Don't attempt everything at once. Introduce one new habit per day—whether it's a morning meditation, an evening wind-down routine, or a new breakfast.

5. **Track Your Progress:** Keep a journal of sleep, mood, and energy levels. This helps you notice improvements beyond the scale.

Transitioning with intention ensures that you won't feel deprived or overwhelmed. Each small step compounds, creating lasting balance over the 28 days.

Daily Rituals for Calming Your Nervous System (Morning + Evening)

Cortisol peaks and dips in a natural rhythm. By syncing your daily routines to this rhythm, you can gently regulate it rather than fight it.

Morning Rituals:

- Start with **deep, slow breaths** for 3–5 minutes before getting out of bed.

- **Hydrate** with a glass of water or warm lemon water to kickstart metabolism.

- Eat a **protein-rich breakfast** with healthy fats and fiber to stabilize blood sugar.

- Step outside or near a window for **natural sunlight exposure**, signaling your body that it's daytime and setting the circadian rhythm.

Evening Rituals:

- Dim lights and reduce screen exposure at least 60 minutes before bed.

- Engage in **mindful reflection**: journal about your day or practice gratitude.

- Enjoy a **light, calming snack** if needed, like almond butter with apple slices or herbal tea.

- Take 5–10 minutes to do **gentle stretches or yoga nidra**, helping muscles relax and cortisol to decrease naturally.

These rituals are simple, yet profoundly effective. They act as anchors in your day, training your nervous system to shift from stress to calm repeatedly.

How to Measure Progress Beyond the Scale

Weight is only one piece of the puzzle. Focusing solely on pounds can be misleading and discouraging. Instead, monitor **holistic progress**:

- **Sleep Quality:** Are you falling asleep faster and waking up more refreshed?

- **Energy Levels:** Do you feel steady energy throughout the day instead of crashing after meals?

- **Mood Stability:** Are irritability, anxiety, or "brain fog" diminishing?

- **Digestive Health:** Is bloating or discomfort less frequent?

- **Mental Clarity:** Are you able to focus longer and recall information more easily?

Keep a small journal. Even noting one positive change daily reinforces progress, motivates adherence, and highlights improvements that the scale alone cannot capture.

Final Thoughts

The 28-day blueprint isn't just a program — it's a **gentle guide back to your body's natural rhythm**. Each week is a layer of support, each daily ritual a tool for calm, and every balanced meal a message of care to your adrenal system.

Remember, transformation is gradual. Celebrate small victories, honor your journey, and give yourself grace on days when stress feels heavier. By following this blueprint, you're not just "detoxing"—you're **reclaiming your energy, focus, and peace**, creating habits that last far beyond these four weeks.

This is your opportunity to reset, rebalance, rebuild, and truly thrive.

Chapter 4

The Science of Stress-Reducing Nutrition

How Blood Sugar and Cortisol Dance Together

Cortisol and blood sugar share a delicate partnership. When blood sugar dips too low, your body perceives it as a stressor, triggering cortisol release to stabilize levels. Conversely, chronic high blood sugar can overstimulate the adrenal glands, causing cortisol imbalances that manifest as fatigue, cravings, and stubborn belly fat.

The key to harmony is **steady energy**. Balanced meals that combine protein, fiber, and healthy fats create a slow, steady release of glucose into your bloodstream. This prevents sharp spikes and crashes, signaling to your body that all is well and keeping cortisol within its natural rhythm.

Practical tip: Pair every carbohydrate with protein or healthy fat. For example, instead of eating plain oatmeal, add almond butter and chia seeds. This not only stabilizes blood sugar but also prolongs satiety and keeps energy levels calm throughout the morning.

The Power of Protein, Fiber, and Healthy Fats for Hormone Harmony

Protein:
Protein is the cornerstone of cortisol balance. Amino

acids—the building blocks of protein—support
neurotransmitter production, which in turn influences
mood and stress resilience. Lean proteins like eggs,
poultry, fish, lentils, and beans also stabilize blood
sugar, reducing the need for cortisol-driven glucose
release.

Fiber:
Fiber slows digestion and maintains steady energy,
reducing spikes in cortisol. Incorporate colorful
vegetables, whole grains, and legumes into your meals.
Fiber also supports gut health, which plays a pivotal role
in hormone regulation. A healthy gut microbiome signals
to your nervous system that your body is safe, lowering
chronic stress responses.

Healthy Fats:
Omega-3s, monounsaturated fats, and plant-based oils
help reduce inflammation and improve adrenal function.
Foods like salmon, avocado, olive oil, walnuts, and
flaxseed not only nourish your cells but also support
mental clarity and mood stability.

Cooking tip: Roast vegetables with olive oil and a
sprinkle of seeds for crunch and added healthy fats. Not
only does this enhance flavor, but it also improves
nutrient absorption, especially fat-soluble vitamins like A,
D, E, and K.

Anti-Inflammatory Meal Planning Made Simple

Inflammation is a hidden driver of cortisol imbalance. The foods you choose every day can either fuel inflammation or soothe it.

Focus on:

- **Anti-inflammatory vegetables:** Spinach, kale, broccoli, bell peppers, zucchini

- **Fruits:** Blueberries, cherries, citrus, pomegranate

- **Proteins:** Fatty fish, pasture-raised poultry, legumes

- **Herbs & spices:** Turmeric, ginger, cinnamon, garlic

Tip: Build your meals like a **rainbow on a plate**. The diversity of colors signals a variety of phytonutrients, antioxidants, and minerals that collectively support adrenal health and reduce oxidative stress.

Meal prep suggestion: Cook a batch of roasted vegetables and quinoa at the start of the week. Combine with lean protein for lunch or dinner, ensuring you always have a nutrient-dense, stress-reducing option ready.

Hydration and Electrolyte Balance for Adrenal Recovery

Your adrenal glands rely on **hydration and electrolytes** to function optimally. Water alone is not enough—sodium, potassium, magnesium, and calcium play key roles in maintaining blood pressure, nerve function, and stress response.

- **Potassium-rich foods:** Sweet potatoes, spinach, bananas

- **Magnesium sources:** Almonds, pumpkin seeds, leafy greens

- **Hydration strategy:** Start your day with water, sip consistently, and consider mineral-rich beverages like coconut water or herbal teas

Practical tip: Instead of relying on caffeine for energy, hydrate first. Dehydration is a hidden cortisol trigger that can exacerbate stress, fatigue, and cravings.

Hidden Cortisol Triggers: Caffeine, Alcohol, Refined Carbs, and Timing Mistakes

Even small lifestyle choices can inadvertently keep cortisol elevated. Awareness is key.

- **Caffeine:** Moderate consumption is fine, but excess, especially later in the day, can delay cortisol decline and disrupt sleep. Pair your coffee with protein or healthy fat to reduce spikes.

- **Alcohol:** Evening alcohol may feel relaxing, but it interferes with deep sleep cycles, increasing morning cortisol. Opt for herbal tea or warm water as a nighttime ritual.

- **Refined carbs & sugar:** Processed bread, pastries, and sugary drinks create rapid glucose spikes, forcing cortisol to act as a stabilizer. Replace with whole grains and fiber-rich alternatives.

- **Timing mistakes:** Eating large meals late at night or skipping meals can confuse your circadian rhythm and stress response. Space meals evenly, with balanced macros, to keep cortisol steady.

Final Thoughts

Nutrition is more than sustenance—it's a powerful ally in your journey toward cortisol balance. Every choice you make feeds not just your body, but your hormones, energy, and mental clarity. By pairing protein with fiber, including healthy fats, and staying mindful of hidden triggers, you create meals that are both delicious and transformative.

Remember: nourishing your body doesn't have to feel restrictive. Flavor, variety, and satisfaction are part of the plan. Think of each meal as an opportunity to restore balance, reset your adrenal system, and take a step closer to thriving.

With the science of stress-reducing nutrition as your foundation, you're empowered to approach the 28-day plan with confidence, knowing that each bite you take supports harmony from the inside out.

Chapter 5

Pantry Makeover & Smart Shopping Guide

Stocking Your Kitchen for Cortisol Balance

A cortisol-friendly diet starts long before the first bite—it begins with your pantry. Your kitchen should be a supportive environment, filled with ingredients that make stress-reducing meals easy, quick, and satisfying.

Start by **evaluating your current pantry**: remove processed snacks, sugary beverages, artificial additives, and foods that trigger blood sugar spikes. The goal is to replace them with nutrient-dense, adrenal-supportive ingredients that nourish your body while keeping cortisol levels steady.

Once your pantry is stocked with these essentials, creating balanced meals will feel natural, effortless, and even exciting. Cooking becomes a joy instead of a chore, and you'll feel more in control of your health journey.

Essential Pantry Staples (Brand-Neutral Examples)

Here are the core staples every cortisol-friendly kitchen should have:

Proteins:

- Lentils, chickpeas, black beans (canned or dried)

- Canned tuna or salmon (in water or olive oil)

- Quinoa, farro, and other whole grains

- Eggs and nut butters for convenience

Healthy Fats:

- Extra virgin olive oil

- Coconut oil for high-heat cooking

- Avocados

- Nuts (almonds, walnuts, cashews) and seeds (chia, flax, pumpkin)

Vegetables & Fruits:

- Frozen or fresh spinach, kale, broccoli, cauliflower

- Sweet potatoes, zucchini, carrots

- Berries (blueberries, raspberries), apples, citrus fruits

Herbs & Spices:

- Turmeric, cinnamon, ginger, garlic, basil, oregano, rosemary

- Sea salt, black pepper, paprika

Pantry Basics:

- Rolled oats or steel-cut oats

- Brown rice or wild rice

- Whole-grain bread or wraps

- Herbal teas (chamomile, peppermint, rooibos)

Hydration & Miscellaneous:

- Mineral-rich water or coconut water

- Apple cider vinegar for salad dressings

- Plant-based milk (unsweetened almond, oat, or soy milk)

Tip: Keep your pantry visually organized and easily accessible. When ingredients are in plain sight, you're more likely to use them creatively in meals rather than resorting to quick, processed options.

Reading Labels Like a Nutritionist

Even with the best intentions, many packaged foods hide stress-inducing ingredients. Becoming a savvy label reader is critical.

1. **Check Sugar Content:** Avoid products with added sugar, high-fructose corn syrup, or multiple words ending in "-ose."

2. **Look at Ingredients List Length:** The shorter and simpler, the better. If you don't recognize most of the ingredients, it's likely processed.

3. **Identify Hidden Additives:** Artificial flavors, preservatives, and colorings can spike cortisol. Stick to whole foods as much as possible.

4. **Assess Sodium Levels:** Too much sodium may affect blood pressure and adrenal health. Use sea salt sparingly.

5. **Understand Fat Types:** Look for healthy fats like olive oil, avocado oil, and nuts. Avoid trans fats or hydrogenated oils.

Practical tip: When in doubt, compare products side by side and choose the one with fewer ingredients, more fiber, and natural sources of protein and fat.

How to Prep a Week's Worth of Meals in Two Hours

Meal prep doesn't have to be overwhelming. With a strategic approach, you can prepare **seven days of stress-reducing meals in just two hours**.

Step 1: Plan Your Menu

- Choose simple breakfasts, lunches, and dinners from your 28-day blueprint recipes.

- Include a variety of proteins, vegetables, and healthy fats to keep meals satisfying and balanced.

Step 2: Batch Cook Basics

- Roast vegetables like broccoli, carrots, and zucchini in one sheet pan.

- Cook a large batch of grains such as quinoa or brown rice.

- Prepare proteins like baked chicken, lentil stew, or boiled eggs.

Step 3: Portion and Store

- Use glass containers for easy access and portion control.

- Store breakfast components, lunch salads, and dinner bases separately to mix and match flavors.

Step 4: Flavor and Finish

- Pre-chop herbs, dressings, and sauces.

- Keep spices and condiments ready to elevate meals quickly.

Step 5: Maintain Freshness

- Freeze items you won't eat within 3–4 days.

- Rotate prepped meals throughout the week to avoid boredom.

Practical tip: Label containers with dates to ensure freshness and minimize waste. A well-organized prep station reduces decision fatigue and keeps your cortisol-friendly routine consistent.

Tips for Eating Well on a Budget

Eating nutrient-dense meals doesn't need to drain your wallet. With planning and smart shopping, you can support your adrenal health without overspending.

1. **Buy in Bulk:** Whole grains, nuts, seeds, and legumes are cheaper in larger quantities and store well.

2. **Embrace Frozen Produce:** Frozen vegetables and fruits are often more affordable, nutritionally equivalent to fresh, and convenient for quick meals.

3. **Seasonal Shopping:** Choose fruits and vegetables in season—they're more flavorful, nutrient-rich, and lower in cost.

4. **Cook at Home:** Pre-packaged meals and restaurant options are typically higher in sodium and hidden sugars. Home-cooked meals give you control over every ingredient.

5. **Plan Leftovers Strategically:** Transform dinner into lunch the next day, or turn roasted veggies into a frittata or grain bowl.

Practical tip: Make a grocery list before every trip. Sticking to a list prevents impulse buys of processed snacks or sugar-laden foods that trigger cortisol spikes.

Final Thoughts

A well-stocked pantry is your secret weapon for long-term cortisol balance. When your kitchen is organized, ingredients are wholesome, and meals are prepped ahead, eating well becomes effortless.

Remember: **a cortisol-friendly kitchen is a happy kitchen**. The combination of smart shopping, batch cooking, and mindful ingredient choices makes it easy to stay on track, nourish your body, and feel empowered every time you open the fridge.

With your pantry optimized, you're now ready to explore **Chapter 6 — Breakfasts to Calm and Energize**, where we dive into **8 delicious, cortisol-supporting breakfast recipes** that will kickstart your mornings with energy, focus, and satisfaction.

Chapter 6

<u>The Cortisol Detox Recipes</u>

Welcome to the heart of your cortisol-reset journey — the recipes! This chapter is carefully crafted to **nourish your body, balance your hormones, and delight your taste buds**. Every recipe is designed with precision to **stabilize blood sugar, reduce inflammation, and support adrenal health**, while remaining easy, affordable, and enjoyable.

From vibrant breakfasts that set a calm tone for the day to satisfying lunches, restorative dinners, and indulgent yet balanced snacks and desserts, these dishes will help you **feel energized, focused, and relaxed**.

Each recipe includes **prep & cook time, portion size, nutritional breakdown, and simple preparation steps**, with optional variations for vegan and gluten-free preferences.

Cooking becomes a joyful experience when it's **approachable, flavorful, and purposeful**. Let's dive in!

Morning Calm

Breakfasts That Lower Morning Cortisol

1. Omega-Boost Chia Porridge

- **Prep & Cook Time:** 5 min prep, 5 min soak

- **Portion Size:** 1 serving

- **Nutritional Breakdown:** 320 cal | Protein 12g | Fat 15g | Carbs 35g | Key Nutrients: Omega-3s, Fiber, Magnesium

Ingredients:

- 3 tbsp chia seeds

- 1 cup unsweetened almond milk

- 1 tsp ground flaxseed

- ½ tsp cinnamon

- ½ cup fresh berries

- 1 tsp maple syrup (optional)

Method:

1. Mix chia seeds, almond milk, flaxseed, and cinnamon in a bowl.

2. Let soak 5 minutes; refrigerate 10–15 min for a creamier texture.

3. Top with berries and drizzle maple syrup.

Tips: Swap berries for diced apple or pear.

---

2. Almond & Banana Overnight Oats

- **Prep & Cook Time:** 5 min prep, overnight soak

- **Portion Size:** 1 serving

- **Nutritional Breakdown:** 330 cal | Protein 11g | Fat 14g | Carbs 40g | Key Nutrients: Magnesium, Fiber, Healthy Fats

Ingredients:

- ½ cup rolled oats

- 1 cup almond milk

- 1 small banana, mashed

- 1 tbsp almond butter

- ½ tsp cinnamon

Method:

1. Mix all ingredients in a jar.

2. Refrigerate overnight.

3. Stir in the morning and enjoy.

Tips: Add cacao nibs for antioxidants.

---

3. Avocado-Egg Power Toast

- **Prep & Cook Time:** 5 min

- **Portion Size:** 1 serving

- **Nutritional Breakdown:** 350 cal | Protein 14g | Fat 22g | Carbs 28g | Key Nutrients: Monounsaturated fats, B-Vitamins

Ingredients:

- 1 slice whole-grain bread

- ½ avocado, mashed

- 1 poached egg

- Pinch black pepper and smoked paprika

Method:

1. Toast bread.

2. Spread avocado and top with egg.

3. Season and enjoy.

Tips: Add cherry tomatoes for antioxidants.

---

4. Spinach & Mushroom Frittata

- **Prep & Cook Time:** 10 min prep, 15 min cook

- **Portion Size:** 1 serving

- **Nutritional Breakdown:** 280 cal | Protein 18g | Fat 18g | Carbs 8g | Key Nutrients: B-Vitamins, Iron

Ingredients:

- 2 eggs

- 1 cup spinach

- ½ cup mushrooms

- 1 tsp olive oil

* Salt & pepper

Method:

1. Preheat the oven 350°F.

2. Sauté veggies, pour in eggs.

3. Bake for 12–15 min.

Tips: Add bell peppers for extra flavor.

---

5. Quinoa & Berry Breakfast Bowl

* **Prep & Cook Time:** 10 min

* **Portion Size:** 1 serving

* **Nutritional Breakdown:** 310 cal | Protein 10g | Fat 9g | Carbs 50g | Key Nutrients: Fiber, Antioxidants

Ingredients:

* ½ cup cooked quinoa

* ½ cup mixed berries

* 1 tbsp pumpkin seeds

- ½ tsp cinnamon

Method:

1. Mix quinoa, berries, pumpkin seeds.

2. Sprinkle cinnamon.

3. Serve warm or cold.

Tips: Swap quinoa for oats if desired.

---

6. Coconut & Blueberry Smoothie Bowl

- **Prep & Cook Time:** 5 min

- **Portion Size:** 1 serving

- **Nutritional Breakdown:** 280 cal | Protein 10g | Fat 12g | Carbs 35g | Key Nutrients: Fiber, Healthy Fats

Ingredients:

- 1 cup coconut milk

- ½ cup blueberries

- 1 tbsp shredded coconut

- ½ tsp cinnamon

- 1 tsp chia seeds

Method:

1. Blend milk and blueberries.

2. Top with coconut and chia.

Tips: Add protein powder if desired.

---

7. Sweet Potato & Kale Breakfast Hash

- **Prep & Cook Time:** 10 min prep, 15 min cook

- **Portion Size:** 1 serving

- **Nutritional Breakdown:** 300 cal | Protein 12g | Fat 14g | Carbs 32g | Key Nutrients: Vitamin A, Fiber

Ingredients:

- 1 small sweet potato

- 1 cup kale

- 1 tsp olive oil

- Salt, pepper, paprika

Method:

1. Sauté sweet potato, add kale, season, and serve.

2. Optional: top with poached egg.

Midday Focus

Lunches to Sustain Energy

1. Citrus-Ginger Salmon Bowl

- **Prep & Cook Time:** 15 min

- **Portion Size:** 1

- **Nutritional Breakdown:** 400 cal | Protein 28g | Fat 18g | Carbs 30g | Key Nutrients: Omega-3s, Vitamin C

Ingredients:

- 4 oz salmon

- 1 cup cooked quinoa

- ½ cup steamed broccoli

- Citrus-ginger dressing

Method:

1. Grill salmon, steam veggies.

2. Serve over quinoa, drizzle dressing.

Tips: Swap salmon for tofu.

---

2. Lentil & Spinach Power Salad

- **Prep & Cook Time:** 10 min

- **Portion Size:** 1

- **Nutritional Breakdown:** 350 cal | Protein 15g | Fat 10g | Carbs 45g | Key Nutrients: Fiber, Iron

Ingredients:

- 1 cup cooked lentils

- 1 cup spinach

- ½ cup diced cucumber

- Lemon vinaigrette

Method:

1. Mix ingredients, drizzle dressing.

2. Serve chilled or room temperature.

---

3. Turkey & Avocado Lettuce Wraps

- **Prep & Cook Time:** 10 min

- **Portion Size:** 1–2 wraps

- **Nutritional Breakdown:** 360 cal | Protein 25g | Fat 18g | Carbs 20g | Key Nutrients: Protein, Monounsaturated fats

Ingredients:

- 4 oz sliced turkey

- 2 large lettuce leaves

- ½ avocado

- Tomato slices

Method:

1. Fill lettuce with ingredients, roll, and serve.

---

4. Mediterranean Chickpea Bowl

- **Prep & Cook Time:** 15 min

- **Portion Size:** 1

- **Nutritional Breakdown:** 380 cal | Protein 16g | Fat 12g | Carbs 50g | Key Nutrients: Fiber, Protein

Ingredients:

- 1 cup chickpeas

- ½ cup cherry tomatoes

- ¼ cup olives

- Drizzle olive oil

Method:

1. Mix ingredients, season, and enjoy.

5. Chicken & Roasted Veggie Quinoa Bowl

- **Prep & Cook Time:** 20 min

- **Portion Size:** 1

- **Nutritional Breakdown:** 420 cal | Protein 30g | Fat 15g | Carbs 40g

Ingredients:

- 4 oz grilled chicken

- 1 cup roasted vegetables

- ½ cup cooked quinoa

Method:

1. Roast veggies, grill chicken, and serve with quinoa.

---

6. Spinach, Mushroom & Egg Wrap

- **Prep & Cook Time:** 10 min

- **Portion Size:** 1

- **Nutritional Breakdown:** 320 cal | Protein 18g | Fat 14g | Carbs 28g

Ingredients:

- 1 whole-grain wrap

- 2 eggs, scrambled

- ½ cup spinach

- ½ cup mushrooms

Method:

1. Scramble eggs with spinach and mushrooms.

2. Wrap and serve.

---

7. Zucchini Noodles with Pesto & Shrimp

- **Prep & Cook Time:** 15 min

- **Portion Size:** 1

- **Nutritional Breakdown:** 380 cal | Protein 25g | Fat 16g | Carbs 30g

Ingredients:

- 1 cup zucchini noodles

- 4 oz shrimp

- 2 tbsp pesto (nut-free optional)

Method:

1. Sauté shrimp, toss with zucchini noodles and pesto.

Evening Reset

Dinners to Soothe Stress

1. Lemon-Herb Baked Salmon with Asparagus

- **Prep & Cook Time:** 20 min

- **Portion Size:** 1

- **Nutritional Breakdown:** 420 cal | Protein 28g | Fat 18g | Carbs 25g

Ingredients & Method: Bake salmon with lemon, herbs, and asparagus at 375°F for 15–20 min.

2. Quinoa & Vegetable Stir-Fry with Tofu

- **Prep & Cook Time:** 15 min

- **Portion Size:** 1

- **Nutritional Breakdown:** 380 cal | Protein 20g | Fat 12g | Carbs 45g

Method: Sauté mixed veggies and tofu, served over quinoa.

3. Turkey & Sweet Potato Skillet

- **Prep & Cook Time:** 20 min

- **Portion Size:** 1

- **Nutritional Breakdown:** 400 cal | Protein 28g | Fat 15g | Carbs 35g

Method: Cook turkey and sweet potato together, season with paprika.

4. Coconut-Curry Chickpea & Spinach Stew

- **Prep & Cook Time:** 15 min

- **Portion Size:** 1

- **Nutritional Breakdown:** 360 cal | Protein 14g |
  Fat 14g | Carbs 45g

Method: Sauté chickpeas, spinach, and curry in coconut
milk.

---

5. Lemon-Garlic Shrimp & Broccoli

- **Prep & Cook Time:** 15 min

- **Portion Size:** 1

- **Nutritional Breakdown:** 370 cal | Protein 25g |
  Fat 15g | Carbs 28g

Method: Sauté shrimp with garlic, served with steamed
broccoli.

---

6. Baked Cod with Zucchini & Cherry Tomatoes

- **Prep & Cook Time:** 20 min

- **Portion Size:** 1

- **Nutritional Breakdown:** 360 cal | Protein 28g | Fat 14g | Carbs 28g | Key Nutrients: Omega-3s, Vitamin C, Fiber

Ingredients:

- 4 oz cod fillet

- 1 cup zucchini, sliced

- ½ cup cherry tomatoes

- 1 tsp olive oil

- Lemon juice, garlic, herbs

Method:

1. Preheat the oven to 375°F (190°C).

2. Toss zucchini and cherry tomatoes with olive oil, garlic, and herbs.

3. Place cod on top and drizzle lemon juice.

4. Bake for 15–20 minutes until the fish flakes easily.

5. Serve warm, optionally with a small side of quinoa or brown rice.

Tips: Swap cod with halibut or tilapia for variety.

7. Mediterranean Chicken & Veggie Tray Bake

- **Prep & Cook Time:** 20 min prep, 30 min cook

- **Portion Size:** 1

- **Nutritional Breakdown:** 410 cal | Protein 32g | Fat 16g | Carbs 30g | Key Nutrients: Protein, Vitamin C, Fiber

Ingredients:

- 4 oz chicken breast

- 1 cup mixed bell peppers and zucchini

- 1 tsp olive oil

- Garlic, herbs, and lemon slices

Method:

1. Preheat the oven to 400°F (200°C).

2. Arrange chicken and veggies on a tray, drizzle olive oil, season.

3. Roast 25–30 minutes until chicken is cooked through.

4. Serve hot with lemon wedges.

Tips: Add olives for extra Mediterranean flavor.

Sly Snacks & Smooth Elixirs –

Quick Bites & Drinks for Balance

1. Golden Turmeric Latte

- **Prep & Cook Time:** 5 min

- **Portion Size:** 1 cup

- **Nutritional Breakdown:** 120 cal | Protein 2g | Fat 6g | Carbs 10g | Key Nutrients: Anti-inflammatory curcumin, Magnesium

Ingredients:

- 1 cup unsweetened almond milk

- ½ tsp turmeric

- ¼ tsp cinnamon

- 1 tsp honey (optional)

Method:

1. Heat almond milk gently.

2. Stir in turmeric, cinnamon, and honey.

3. Serve warm.

---

2. Almond & Cocoa Energy Bites

- **Prep & Cook Time:** 10 min

- **Portion Size:** 2–3 bites

- **Nutritional Breakdown:** 150 cal | Protein 5g | Fat 10g | Carbs 12g | Key Nutrients: Magnesium, Fiber, Protein

Ingredients:

- ¼ cup almond butter

- 2 tbsp cocoa powder

- 2 tbsp rolled oats

- 1 tsp honey

Method:

1. Mix ingredients, form small balls.

2. Refrigerate 10 min before serving.

---

3. Avocado & Cucumber Smoothie

- **Prep & Cook Time:** 5 min

- **Portion Size:** 1 cup

- **Nutritional Breakdown:** 180 cal | Protein 3g | Fat 12g | Carbs 18g | Key Nutrients: Healthy fats, Hydration, Fiber

Ingredients:

- ½ avocado

- 1 cup cucumber

- 1 cup coconut water

- Juice of ½ lime

Method:

1. Blend all ingredients until smooth.

2. Serve chilled.

---

4. Cinnamon-Spiced Apple Chips

- **Prep & Cook Time:** 10 min prep, 30 min bake

- **Portion Size:** 1 serving

- **Nutritional Breakdown:** 120 cal | Protein 0g | Fat 0g | Carbs 30g | Key Nutrients: Fiber, Polyphenols

Ingredients:

- 1 apple, thinly sliced

- ½ tsp cinnamon

Method:

1. Preheat the oven to 200°F (90°C).

2. Spread apple slices, sprinkle cinnamon.

3. Bake 25–30 min until crisp.

---

5. Spinach & Pineapple Smoothie

- **Prep & Cook Time:** 5 min

- **Portion Size:** 1 cup

- **Nutritional Breakdown:** 160 cal | Protein 2g | Fat 1g | Carbs 35g | Key Nutrients: Vitamin C, Antioxidants

Ingredients:

- 1 cup spinach

- ½ cup pineapple

- 1 cup water or coconut water

Method:

1. Blend until smooth.

2. Serve immediately.

---

6. Dark Chocolate & Almond Clusters

- **Prep & Cook Time:** 10 min

- **Portion Size:** 2–3 clusters

- **Nutritional Breakdown:** 150 cal | Protein 4g | Fat 10g | Carbs 12g | Key Nutrients: Magnesium, Healthy fats, Antioxidants

Ingredients:

- ¼ cup almonds
- 2 tbsp dark chocolate (70%+)
- Pinch sea salt

Method:

1. Melt chocolate, stir in almonds.
2. Drop clusters onto parchment paper.
3. Chill 10–15 min before serving.

Final Thoughts – Enjoy Cooking with Confidence and Creativity

Congratulations! You now have a full arsenal of **delicious, cortisol-lowering recipes** to guide you through the 28-day reset. Each meal, snack, and elixir is designed to **nourish your body, stabilize your energy, and restore hormonal balance**.

Remember: **cooking is not just about following instructions—it's about exploring flavors, experimenting with seasonal produce, and finding joy in nourishing yourself**. Swap ingredients, try new spices, and share these recipes with friends and family to make your journey even more enjoyable.

Your kitchen is your sanctuary, your meals are your medicine, and with these recipes, you're set to transform not only your **hormonal health** but your **overall well-being**.

Chapter 7

<u>The 28-Day Meal Plan</u>

Welcome to the heart of your cortisol reset journey! Here, you'll find a **practical, easy-to-follow, and scientifically designed 28-day plan** that combines all the knowledge and recipes we've covered in the previous chapters. This is more than just a meal schedule—it's your **personal roadmap to hormonal balance, reduced stress, and renewed energy**.

Whether you're a busy professional, a parent juggling responsibilities, or someone who has struggled with fatigue and stubborn weight gain, this plan is crafted to **simplify your life while nourishing your body**. You no longer have to wonder what to eat or when—the plan guides you step by step.

Every week has been designed around **four key principles**:

1. **Reset:** Stabilize cortisol with nutrient-rich, easy-to-digest foods.

2. **Rebalance:** Strengthen adrenal function and improve energy levels.

3. **Rebuild:** Support metabolism, muscle repair, and sustained focus.

4. **Thrive:** Solidify healthy habits, encourage creativity in the kitchen, and maintain hormonal harmony.

Each day's plan includes:

- **Breakfast** – Energizing meals to lower morning cortisol.

- **Lunch** – Balanced lunches that sustain energy and focus.

- **Dinner** – Relaxing meals that support evening reset and restful sleep.

- **Snack** – Quick bites or beverages for balance between meals.

Weekly Layout

Week 1 — Reset

Goal: Stabilize cortisol levels and introduce balanced nutrition. Focus on anti-inflammatory foods, high fiber, and quality protein.
 Weekly Focus: Sleep hygiene, hydration, gentle movement.

Sample Daily Menu:

Day 1

- **Breakfast:** Omega-Boost Chia Porridge (Prep: 5 min, Cook: 5 min)

- **Lunch:** Citrus-Ginger Salmon Bowl with Quinoa (Prep: 10 min, Cook: 20 min)

- **Dinner:** Baked Cod with Zucchini & Cherry Tomatoes (Prep: 10 min, Cook: 20 min)

- **Snack:** Almond & Cocoa Energy Bites (Prep: 10 min)

Day 2

- **Breakfast:** Spinach & Mushroom Scramble with Herbs (Prep: 5 min, Cook: 10 min)

- **Lunch:** Mediterranean Chicken & Veggie Tray Bake (Prep: 10 min, Cook: 30 min)

- **Dinner:** Turmeric Coconut Lentil Soup (Prep: 10 min, Cook: 25 min)

- **Snack:** Golden Turmeric Latte (Prep: 5 min)

Continue Days 3–7 with unique combinations from Chapter 6 recipes.

Week 2 — Rebalance

Goal: Enhance adrenal recovery and optimize blood sugar balance.

Weekly Focus: Mindful eating, moderate exercise, morning and evening rituals.

Sample Daily Menu:

Day 8

- **Breakfast:** Avocado & Spinach Smoothie Bowl (Prep: 5 min)

- **Lunch:** Spinach-Quinoa Power Plate with Lemon Dressing (Prep: 10 min)

- **Dinner:** Mediterranean Chicken & Veggie Tray Bake with roasted garlic hummus (Prep: 10 min, Cook: 30 min)

- **Snack:** Cinnamon-Spiced Apple Chips (Prep: 10 min, Cook: 25–30 min)

Day 9

- **Breakfast:** Blueberry-Oat Pancakes with Almond Butter (Prep: 10 min, Cook: 15 min)

- **Lunch:** Citrus-Ginger Salmon Bowl (Prep: 10 min, Cook: 20 min)

- **Dinner:** Baked Cod with Zucchini & Cherry Tomatoes (Prep: 10 min, Cook: 20 min)

- **Snack:** Spinach & Pineapple Smoothie (Prep: 5 min)

Days 10–14 continue with varied recipes from Chapter 6 to keep meals exciting and nutrient-dense.

Week 3 — Rebuild

Goal: Support metabolism, maintain balanced cortisol, and strengthen resilience to stress.
 Weekly Focus: Meal prep for convenience, introduce variety in flavors, continue mindfulness.

Day 15 Example:

- **Breakfast:** Omega-Boost Chia Porridge

- **Lunch:** Spinach-Quinoa Power Plate

- **Dinner:** Turmeric Coconut Lentil Soup

- **Snack:** Dark Chocolate & Almond Clusters

Continue Days 16–21 with thoughtfully rotated recipes to ensure every day feels fresh and satisfying.

Week 4 — Thrive

Goal: Reinforce sustainable habits, explore creative recipes, and solidify energy and sleep improvements.
 Weekly Focus: Reflect, journal progress, enjoy cooking creatively.

Day 22 Example:

- **Breakfast:** Spinach & Mushroom Scramble with Herbs

- **Lunch:** Citrus-Ginger Salmon Bowl

- **Dinner:** Mediterranean Chicken & Veggie Tray Bake

- **Snack:** Almond & Cocoa Energy Bites

Days 23–28: Rotate all Chapter 6 recipes while introducing optional ingredient swaps for variety.

Batch Cooking & Substitutions

- Prepare grains like quinoa, rice, and lentils in **bulk** at the start of each week.

- Roast vegetables in **large batches** to save time.

- Swap proteins: Salmon → Cod → Chicken → Tofu (vegan option).

- Dairy swaps: Almond milk, oat milk, or coconut milk for recipes needing milk.

- Gluten-free options: Use gluten-free oats or pasta as needed.

Weekly Reflection Pages

At the end of each week, take a few moments to **reflect on your progress**. Consider:

- Energy levels (1–10 scale)

- Mood improvements

- Sleep quality (hours and restfulness)

- Notes on cravings or emotional triggers

- Adjustments for the following week

Tip: Use these reflections to fine-tune the plan for your body's unique needs.

Final Thoughts

By the end of this 28-day journey, you will have:

- **A balanced, stress-reducing diet** that supports healthy cortisol levels.

- **A practical approach** to meal prep, shopping, and cooking.

- **Confidence in making substitutions** and keeping meals fresh.

- **A clear roadmap** to maintain hormonal balance beyond the 28 days.

This plan is **science-backed, dietitian-approved, and completely actionable**. Follow it closely, enjoy the meals, and celebrate the small wins—your body, mind, and taste buds will thank you.

With dedication and consistency, you're not just completing a meal plan—you're **resetting your body and reclaiming your energy, focus, and vitality**.

Chapter 8

<u>Lifestyle Strategies to Keep Cortisol in Check</u>

Cortisol isn't just influenced by what you eat—

it's shaped by how you live every single day. While the right nutrition lays the foundation, your **lifestyle habits** determine how well your body can manage stress and maintain balance. This chapter will guide you through **science-backed strategies** that are practical, realistic, and easy to implement, so you can sustain the benefits of your 28-day plan long after it's finished.

---

1. Optimize Sleep for Hormone Harmony

Sleep is your body's **natural reset button**. Poor or inconsistent sleep elevates cortisol, disrupts insulin, and sabotages your energy. Prioritize these habits:

- **Consistent bedtime and wake time:** Going to bed and waking up at the same time every day signals your body to regulate hormone cycles naturally.

- **Create a wind-down routine:** Dim the lights, turn off electronics at least 60 minutes before sleep, and consider calming activities such as journaling, reading, or gentle stretching.

- **Mind your environment:** Keep your bedroom cool, dark, and quiet. Blackout curtains and a white-noise machine can dramatically improve sleep quality.

- **Limit stimulants:** Avoid caffeine after 2 PM and minimize late-night sugar or heavy meals that spike blood sugar.

By making sleep a non-negotiable priority, you allow your body to **repair, recover, and regulate cortisol** effectively.

---

2. Movement That Heals

Exercise is a double-edged sword—it can either reduce or raise cortisol depending on type, intensity, and timing. Focus on:

- **Gentle cardio:** Walking, light jogging, or cycling can reduce stress hormones without overstressing your body.

- **Yoga and stretching:** Practices like yin yoga or restorative stretches help calm the nervous system while improving flexibility and circulation.

- **Resistance training:** Moderate weightlifting or bodyweight exercises support metabolism and build resilience to stress.

- **Mindful movement:** Tai chi, pilates, or even mindful walking combines exercise with mindfulness, helping your body release cortisol naturally.

Tip: Avoid excessively intense workouts late in the evening, as these can spike cortisol and disrupt sleep.

---

3. Breathwork and Relaxation Techniques

Your breath is a powerful tool for **calming the nervous system**. Incorporate these techniques:

- **Box breathing:** Inhale 4 counts, hold 4, exhale 4, hold 4. Repeat for 5 minutes.

- **Diaphragmatic breathing:** Breathe deeply into your belly instead of shallow chest breathing.

- **Mindful pauses:** Take 2–3 minutes during your day to focus on slow, controlled breaths.

These simple practices **activate the parasympathetic nervous system**, signaling your body that it's safe to relax, which **lowers cortisol naturally**.

---

4. Creating Stress-Proof Morning and Evening Routines

Morning: Start your day with intentional habits that support energy and focus.

- Hydrate immediately upon waking (warm water or herbal tea).

- Eat a protein-rich breakfast (see Chapter 6 for examples).

- Engage in a brief movement or stretch routine.

- Set daily intentions or practice gratitude for 5 minutes.

Evening: Signal to your body that it's time to wind down.

- Avoid screens for at least 60 minutes before bed.

- Sip a calming herbal tea like chamomile or lavender.

- Reflect on wins and jot down tomorrow's priorities in a journal.

- Practice gentle stretches or meditation to release tension.

Consistency is key—**your routines are the framework that stabilizes cortisol** and supports long-term wellness.

---

5. Staying Consistent When Life Gets Busy

Even with the best intentions, life can throw curveballs. Here's how to stay on track:

- **Batch prep meals** (see Chapter 7) to ensure you always have cortisol-friendly options on hand.

- **Prioritize micro-moments of relaxation**—even 2 minutes of mindful breathing counts.

- **Set realistic exercise goals:** It's better to move 15–20 minutes daily than skip entirely because you can't fit an hour in.

- **Embrace flexibility:** If one day doesn't go perfectly, simply get back on track the next. Progress is cumulative.

Remember: **small, consistent actions win over perfection**. These habits compound over time, leading to meaningful reductions in cortisol and improvements in your energy, focus, and mood.

Final Thoughts

Lifestyle strategies are **the glue that holds your cortisol reset together**. Nutrition lays the foundation, but your **sleep, movement, stress management, and routines** determine how well your body can maintain balance.

By integrating these strategies with the 28-day meal plan and recipes from earlier chapters, you're not just completing a program—you're **building a sustainable, life-changing lifestyle**. Celebrate every small win, experiment with routines that suit your life, and enjoy the journey.

Tip: Use this chapter as a reference whenever you feel stressed, overwhelmed, or off-track. Return to these practices regularly—they are your blueprint for lasting hormonal harmony and vitality.

Chapter 9

<u>Advanced Strategies & Long-Term Success</u>

Completing your 28-day cortisol reset is a significant achievement, but true transformation happens when you **carry these habits forward into daily life**. This chapter will guide you through advanced strategies that deepen the benefits of your program, help you manage stress long-term, and maintain hormonal balance without feeling deprived or restricted.

---

1. Adaptogens and Supplements: What Works and What Doesn't

Adaptogens are natural compounds that help your body **adapt to stress and support adrenal health**. While many claim miraculous results, it's essential to focus on what's **scientifically supported, safe, and effective**.

- **Ashwagandha:** Supports healthy cortisol levels and stress resilience. Typical dose: 300–500 mg per day.

- **Rhodiola Rosea:** Can improve energy and reduce mental fatigue. Recommended dose:

200–400 mg daily.

- **Holy Basil (Tulsi):** May help calm the nervous system. 300 mg per day is generally safe.

- **Magnesium:** Supports relaxation, sleep, and muscle function. 200–400 mg per day from supplements or food.

Important: Supplements are **not a replacement for a balanced diet or lifestyle habits**. Always consult a healthcare professional before starting new supplements, especially if you take medications or have underlying health conditions.

---

2. Identifying Your Personal Cortisol Triggers

Everyone reacts differently to stress. Understanding your unique triggers allows you to **proactively manage cortisol spikes**:

- **Keep a stress diary:** Note stressful events, foods, sleep patterns, and how you feel each day.

- **Recognize patterns:** Late-night work, high caffeine intake, skipped meals, or conflict with others may trigger spikes.

- **Develop personalized coping strategies:** Swap triggers with calming practices like short walks, journaling, or deep breathing exercises.

Tip: Awareness is power—once you know your triggers, you can respond intentionally rather than react unconsciously.

---

3. Transitioning Out of the 28-Day Plan Into Everyday Living

After completing the reset, it's important to **integrate new habits without feeling restricted**:

- **Rotate recipes and meal plans:** Continue to enjoy the cortisol-friendly dishes from Chapter 6 while incorporating seasonal foods.

- **Flexible scheduling:** Apply morning and evening routines consistently, even if timing shifts slightly on busy days.

- **Mindful indulgence:** Enjoy treats occasionally without guilt. Balance, not perfection, is the goal.

This transition ensures your **hard-earned results are maintained long-term**, not just during the program.

---

4. Emotional Resilience and Mindset Reframing

Stress management is as much about mindset as it is about nutrition. Cultivating emotional resilience helps you **navigate challenges without chronic cortisol spikes**:

- **Practice gratitude:** Begin or end your day listing three things you're thankful for.

- **Cognitive reframing:** Shift perspective from "I must be perfect" to "I'm making progress."

- **Daily micro-breaks:** Small pauses during the day reduce overwhelm and keep you focused.

Building resilience doesn't happen overnight—but small, consistent mindset shifts **protect your health and enhance well-being**.

---

5. How to Maintain Results Without Dieting

The ultimate goal is sustainable lifestyle change, not temporary dieting:

- **Eat for nourishment, not restriction:** Focus on nutrient-dense foods that keep you full, energized, and hormonally balanced.

- **Keep a flexible routine:** Prioritize sleep, movement, and stress management, even when life gets hectic.

- **Celebrate progress, not perfection:** Reflect weekly on wins and improvements in energy, mood, and focus.

- **Stay curious:** Experiment with new cortisol-friendly foods, recipes, and wellness practices to keep your journey enjoyable.

Maintaining your results is **about creating a lifestyle you love**, not punishing your body with rigid rules.

Final Thoughts

This chapter is your guide to **long-term success**, giving you the tools, mindset, and strategies to thrive well beyond the 28-day plan. By combining nutrition, lifestyle habits, mindfulness, and occasional supplementation, you can **keep cortisol balanced, energy high, and stress manageable**—all while enjoying delicious meals and a fulfilling life.

Remember: lasting change comes from **consistency, awareness, and self-compassion**. Celebrate your progress, trust your body, and continue to use this book as a resource whenever you need guidance, motivation, or inspiration.

Conclusion

Your New Beginning

Congratulations! By completing this journey through the **Cortisol Detox Diet Plan**, you have taken **intentional, life-changing steps** toward reclaiming your energy, focus, and wellbeing. This isn't just the end of a 28-day program—it's the **beginning of a healthier, more balanced life**.

Take a moment to reflect on how far you've come. You've explored the science of cortisol, learned to read your body's signals, and incorporated nutrient-rich, stress-supporting meals into your daily routine. Beyond the recipes and meal plans, you've embraced strategies for sleep, mindful movement, breathwork, and emotional resilience. Each small habit you've practiced has **compounded into real progress**, building a foundation for lasting change.

Remember: **balance is not a one-time achievement— it's a lifelong practice**. There will be days when stress creeps in, routines shift, or life feels overwhelming. And that's okay. What matters is your commitment to return to these tools, strategies, and habits with patience, self-compassion, and confidence. Every mindful choice, every nourishing meal, and every intentional breath reinforces your body's ability to regulate cortisol and thrive.

Think of this book as your companion, your guide, and your **source of inspiration whenever you need support**. The journey toward hormonal balance and stress resilience is ongoing, but now, you are equipped to navigate it with knowledge, confidence, and joy.

So go forward with pride. Celebrate your victories, savor every meal, honor your body's needs, and embrace a lifestyle that nurtures both your mind and your body. You have the tools, the guidance, and the wisdom to continue thriving.

Your new beginning starts today. With every choice, every meal, and every mindful moment, you are creating a life of **energy, clarity, and lasting vitality**. The path to balanced living isn't a destination—it's a journey, and you are fully capable of walking it beautifully.